I *am* the Lord who heals you. Exodus 15:26 NKJV

The

Blueprint

To Weigh Loss

The Truth Exposed

SHERELL BROWN

ISBN:1534634509
ISBN-13:9781534634503

3

I *am* the Lord who heals you. Exodus 15:26 NKJV

I *am* the Lord who heals you. Exodus 15:26 NKJV

THE BLUEPRINT TO WEIGHT LOSS

The Truth Exposed

HOW I LOST 100 POUNDS

SHERELL BROWN

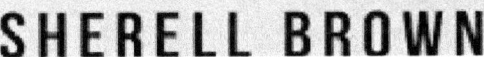
I am the Lord who heals you. Exodus 15:26 NKJV

Acknowledgements

To God be the glory great things he has done. I want to give special thanks to Desmond Brown, my loving husband, who has stood by me through thick and thin (literally). Lord Brown, this would have not been possible without you. Thank you, baby I will always Love you until eternity and beyond. To my two beautiful children, Young Master Seth and Princess Grace, my legacies, Mommy loves you.

To my mother who helped to mold me into the strong woman I am today, from the bottom of my heart thank you and to my Father for your godly example, I love you both. To Sherry Johnson-Deal, my editor, thank you for your unwavering support and to Elle Clarke Media Group for helping me to live beyond my dreams. I am forever grateful.

To my team and support system, Naomi, Kenya and so many others, the people who have nurtured and allowed my gift to blossom, thank you for everything.

I *am* the Lord who heals you. Exodus 15:26 NKJV

About Me

Sherell Brown is "The Diamond Standard" is a category creator in the Health and Wellness arena. Combining a mix of both professional skills and personal experiences that produces results. Sherell has worked with persons from all walks of life helping them to achieve their personal goals.Ultimately creating a better quality of life. She is the C.E.O of Sherell Brown Health Concierge Services, the Publisher of "L.O.S.E" Health & Wellness Magazine, the host of the talk show "Ask Sherell" and Author of The Blueprint To Weight Loss The Truth Revealed. She has spear headed campaigns such as "The Bra Out" a fundraiser design to bring awareness to Breast Cancer in the Island of Abaco, Bahamas, where she also held Aerobic Sessions and went on to launch other campaigns such as "Team No Rolls" and "Lose with Me" She is a sought after Radio Personality .

She is the founder of The War Against Obesity The Cause , where she is teaching people how to eat to live and not to die!She has consulted and motivated thousands of people across the world transforming lives. When speaking with Sherell she will tell you her favorite part of the transformation process is the smile "when the diamond within an individual is unearthed and what they knew was always on the

I *am* the Lord who heals you. Exodus 15:26 NKJV

inside is now glistening on the outside". Most importantly Sherell provides education and tools to help ensure the success of your journey she is dedicated her life to helping other become healthier while teaching them how to reprogram their minds towards food and how you can reset your metabolism. No matter where you are in your health and wellness journey she is there to help you. She also offers limited personal coaching and consulting. With her love for the Lord and her relentless passion, she is ready to serve you.

I *am* the Lord who heals you. Exodus 15:26 NKJV

TABLE OF CONTENTS

I *am* the Lord who heals you. Exodus 15:26 NKJV

Introduction

Metaphorically speaking, to build a house one must first lay the foundation for the house to be structurally sound, this only makes sense. One would not be able to construct a roof without erecting the sides of the house nor assemble the sides of the house without first laying a foundation. Without structural order, the result would not be 'pretty' and the longevity of the structure would be short lived.

The Blueprint To Weight Loss is an interactive guide designed to teach you the principals I applied during my weight loss journey to help you to lay a solid foundation when fulfilling your long-term weight loss goal.

Ahead, you will discover the important yet powerful role the mind plays in the execution of your weight loss goals and how your thoughts ultimately affect your overall success. Subsequently, with a dose of

I *am* the Lord who heals you. Exodus 15:26 NKJV

reality, we learn the numbers with practicals design to stimulate your mind to act. With our minds poised and our numbers in hand, you will be ready to retain the next three simple principals of weight loss.

1. Expose:
2. Expel;
3. Empower.

But just before we get to work I want you to get to know me a little better. In the pages ahead I share with you some of the stories, hurt, pain and shame that help pushed me into my purpose and without further ado lets go to work!!!!

I *am* the Lord who heals you. Exodus 15:26 NKJV

My Journey

"Go from around me!" "Your fat sloppy self!" "Don't come by me, who wants to be around you!" During childhood, these were just some of the phrases I heard ringing in my ears; words that danced to the rhythmic tune of low self-esteem. The continuous verbal beat down that came from family, friends and strangers equaled the total of rejection that manifested in me, both physically and mentally, as you could imagine. Who knew that childhood bullying and the rantings of pre-pubic children could have such lasting effect on a then-fragile self-esteem, this is no fictional story created to entice and entertain you, this was my reality.

By the 6th Grade at age ten years, I remember my physical examination as it was yesterday. After standing on a scale, with the school nurse, doctor and class being present, I was told that I weighed 125 pounds and was overweight. I was a fat kid; this is what the kids who surrounded me translated 'overweight' to mean. I then went on to high school thinking and rejoicing, saying yes to a fresh start; but it only got worse. Realizing now that school back then was like a jungle. Only the strong survived, and I was the weakling. People laughed mocked and called me names. A foul tradition that

12

had been passed down for generations; "if I shine the light on you, maybe you won't see the dirt on me." I had no quick comeback nor witty responses. Most days I just tolerated it until I started to fight back using my own F---- bombs. But the truth is, talking back did not make me feel any better or diminish the hurt and embarrassment that I felt inside.

By the 12th grade, I was nearing a whopping 200 lbs. Starring the freedom of graduation in the face' wide-eyed and eager to run for my life; to have a life or feel like I existed in this life. The psychological scars were now deeply rooted, and the fragile child had now become a woman; now motivated by what once haunted her. Freedom never looked so good. The curves that once brought me so much anguish now brought me more than my fair share of attention. So as you can imagine, I embraced it all. I became obsessed with the gym. Eating and sleeping, aerobics, the wooden gloss glazed floor became my place of solitude. Even in a crowded room, I felt a release like none other. I was finally home and at peace with myself. Fast forwarded, I went on and lived happily ever after the end.

LOL Not just yet! I got married. Then joined the Police Force Academy on the island where I lived at the time and the "F" word launched it's assault on me again during the recruitment process. I was told

13

over and over I was overweight; however, I passed my physical and was permitted to join the academy. I will never forget the first day I met my physical instructor. He said, " not a day I want to see you walking, as a matter of fact, whenever I see you RUN." That was how I spent the next six months, running, motivated by fear, fear of being less than my counterparts.

So I pushed myself twice as hard, and my body turned into a lean machine, well lean, I was a part of C squad 2007. We were 30 strong and known as the running squad, a crazy but determined bunch of people. But it was this group of people that helped to pull me through. I can still remember early morning runs when I would drop behind and Rio, Nabbie or Richie would drop back with me and say come on" Big Mama" as they affectionately called me, saying you can do it and as sure as day, we made it. I can still remember sitting on the floor in the female dormitory with my "squaddies." "THE SHE UNIT" we called ourselves laughing at how one of our instructors came in at 3 am saying " I come like a thief in the night." Laughter filled the hallways as someone asked if he was Jesus. And oh how I can still remember standing proudly on graduation day thanking the Lord that the weight did not beat me for I had made It.

I Then went on to have in the years to come to have

two beautiful children who I love dearly. But along with the love came the pounds, depression, and the low self-esteem. Feelings, emotions, and memories that I thought I had buried had become unearthed coupled with being in a working environment that I no longer desired. My life felt like it was caving in around me; the internal struggle began to show on the outside. There were days I lacked the desire even to groom myself. Nobody knew! Then when I thought life could not get any worse, I hit rock bottom. A medical attack hit my family affecting my husband; I was told that he had Leukemia or a form of Cancer. My then 12-week old daughter had pneumonia, and my son had to be assessed for signs of Autism. The stress of all of this overwhelmed me. No one knew I was having shortness of breath and tightness in my chest; my concern was for my family.

One day during morning prayer, I awoke to hear a loud voice telling me to run, run, run. I was in such fear; I got up and did just that. I ran for the first time in more than five years. While running that same still, the voice told me that I was going to have a heart attack, to confirm my thoughts, I visited the doctor, and the report was not so good. I knew that it was God trying to save my life. I then started running daily at a pace that would be considered a fast walk.

I *am* the Lord who heals you. Exodus 15:26 NKJV

Starting this journey, the last time I went on the scale I weighed 320 pounds In which I had gained from my second pregnancy. As you could imagine, I was less than excited, but motivated by the fact that death could be closer than I thought.

Through the process, I did not only deal with feelings of rejection, low self-esteem, and jealousy at one point. I flirted with suicidal thoughts thinking I should just die. Life had become hard, and it looked like there was no way out but then came my deliverance. Comforting words that came through a stranger reminded me that I was not in this fight alone. God had heard my prayers and restoration had come. I sobbed. This stranger 'read my mail.' She could not possibly know the hurt, struggle and pain I felt and endured. Then one by one thing's started to turn around.

My husband became well, my daughter miraculously healed and my son more energetic than ever. The weight began to fall off, and the inward reflection of myself began to change, then the outside started to fall in line. Through the journey, I had to disconnect myself from the lies and ties from my youth. The poison that I came in agreement with that was contrary to the truth, understanding that self-talk is important; learning that what you believe to be true will come true. When I changed my self-talk, I changed my life! An

I *am* the Lord who heals you. Exodus 15:26 NKJV

old antic says "stick and stones will break my bones, but words will never hurt me," I determined that that was a lie.

Words can hurt you, but you ultimately determine what you chose to believe. I chose to live and have an abundant life and you to can do the same.

I *am* the Lord who heals you. Exodus 15:26 NKJV

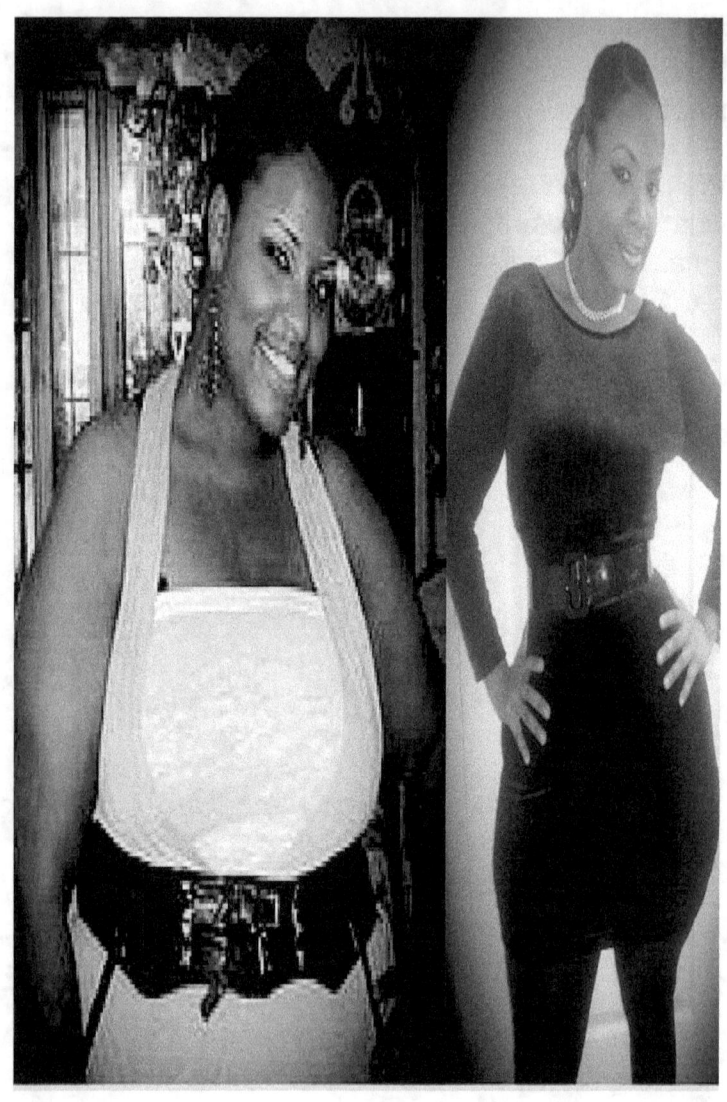

I *am* the Lord who heals you. Exodus 15:26 NKJV

Step One
Your Mind Does Matter

The Bible declares, "As a man thinketh so is he." The mind and its connection to action and manifestation have been under investigation from since time began. At present, one thing is sure - the ability to achieve any goal starts in the mind.

Victory or defeat in any task in life is played out mentally before manifesting physically. This principal applies to weight loss just as it applies to the construction of a building. You must first visualize the end result and then construct a detail plan to achieve the masterpiece.

Before constructing a building, you would first request that the architect drafts a blueprint of the completed project, what I would call the 'physical manifestation.'

Once in view, you would be able to have a clear picture of the finished product and the steps required to complete it. With this visualization, there is an internal excitement which enables an external movement i.e energy generated which would prompt you to action.

For example, you are cleaning out an old cabinet at

19

home, and you stumble across a few old photos. Your jaw drops at the site of a thinner you. Almost instantly you do a 'self-check' realizing you are not where you would like to be physically. That photo can now serve as a blueprint for your desired physique or the end result. However, most persons do not progress beyond the visualization stage. Just as constructing a house is a process, so is weight loss. After the idealization and visualization stage comes preparation; which is where the fight is lost for most persons. That is to say; they have the desire to lose weight and to become healthier, or they can generate a mental picture of their desired weight but somewhere between the preparation and manifestation stages they fall short.

Well, in the coming chapters, we will outline fundamental principals that I implemented in the preparation stage that will help to facilitate the manifestation. Sure enough, the rest is up to you.

I *am* the Lord who heals you. Exodus 15:26 NKJV

Practical Exercise
Breaking Down the Mental Blocks

Your mind is a critical factor in your weight loss journey. Yes, it's a journey, not a sprint. Your body will not transform overnight, but after the consistent daily effort, you will undoubtedly yield results. But first, do you believe that you can attain your weight-loss goal or are you defeated before you have even begun?

For our first exercise, we are going to dispel the lies that you have told yourself about losing weight. You know the lies like I am too fat. I am just big boned. Obesity runs in my family. Nothing will help me. Yes, those lies.

You will need a black pen and a red pen in this first section

1._____
2. _____
3. _____
4._____
5. _____

I *am* the Lord who heals you. Exodus 15:26 NKJV

Step Two
Reality Check

For most of the persons, I have worked with, this stage of the process has been one of the toughest 'pill to swallow'. It forces you to address the truth about where you are and gives you a clear picture of the distance you have to go.

When constructing a building, the next step after drafting your blueprint, in many instances, is inspecting the site where the building would be erected. It is during this stage that the land is cleared i.e. unwanted trees and debris are removed, and the marking is put in place for the foundation to be poured.

Just like the body, we begin to inspect ourselves, removing all assumptions and making assessments of where we are so that we can prepare to lay the foundation that will aid us in our journey.

I *am* the Lord who heals you. Exodus 15:26 NKJV

Practical Exercise

Now with a red pen, write down your goals as it relates to the previous section this is your visualization, your blueprint, your destination. With a black pen fill in the correct answers below. This is your starting point, your marker on the ground, your "I have had enough!"

Age:_____

Sex:_____

Current Weight:_____

Hight:_____

Weight:_____

Hips:_____

Thighs:_____

Arms:_____

Chest:_____

now base on your answer from the previous section, we are going to calculate your Basal Metabolic Rate (BMR) which according to Wikipedia is the minimal amount of energy your body expends per unit at rest. In a nutshell, it is the number of calories your body needs to function to perform activities such as breathing and cell growth.

According to Understanding Metabolism: What Determines Your BMR ... (n.d.). Retrieved from http://www.fitday.com/fitness-articles/nutrition/understanding-metabolism-what-d, your Basal Metabolic Rate (BMR) also affects the rate at which you burn calories and ultimately whether you maintain, gain, or lose weight. Your basal metabolic rate accounts for about 60% to 75% of the calories you burn every day.

Several factors influence it;
For example:
BMR Calculation for Women Imperial
BMR= 655.1 + (4.35 x weight in pounds) + (4.7 x height in inches)- (4.7 x ages in years

Now base on your answer from the previous section, we are going to calculate your Basal Metabolic Rate (BMR) which according to Wikipedia is the minimal amount of energy your body expends per unit at rest. In a nutshell, it is the number of calories your body needs to function to perform activities such as breathing and cell growth. Our Basal Metabolic Rate (BMR) also affects the rate at which you burn calories and ultimately whether you maintain, gain, or lose weight. Your basal metabolic rate accounts for about 60% to 75% of the calories you burn every day.

No am not asking you to perform this equation. Thanks to modern technology the answer is at the click of a button, however, this solution is imperative to your success. With a search engine of your choice type in BMR calculator and learn your number. It will tell you the number of calories you need daily to consume to achieve your desired goal in the amount of time. Your foundation is now laid, and your blueprint is now taking shape.

I *am* the Lord who heals you. Exodus 15:26 NKJV

Step Three
Expose The Lie

Now let's get into the thick of things. The truth is there is no secret to losing weight. It is not a mystical illusion. It is the result of calculated logical steps executed over a period that will give you the desired results. Weight loss occurs two ways:

One, by way of exercise; by burning more calories than you consume. Tow by decreasing your caloric intake.

The first method, exercise, requires you to burn more calories than you consume. Most people found the best success when they combined the two.

The second way is to reduce your calorie intake is by changing your diet.

According to Counting calories: Get back to weight-loss basics - Mayo ... (n.d.). Retrieved from http://www.mayoclinic.org/healthy-lifestyle/weight-loss/in-depth/calories/art-20 , Your weight is a balancing act, but the equation is simple: If you eat more calories than you burn, you gain weight.

Because 3,500 calories equal about 1 pound (0.45

I *am* the Lord who heals you. Exodus 15:26 NKJV

kilogram) of fat, you need to burn 3,500 calories more than you take in to lose 1 pound.

So, in general, if you cut 500 calories from your typical diet each day, you'd lose about 1 pound a week (500 calories x 7 days = 3,500 calories). It isn't quite this simple, however, and you usually lose a combination of fat, lean tissue, and water. Also, because of changes that occur in the body as a result of weight loss, you may need to decrease calories further to continue weight loss.

Calorie reduction is a fundamental principle of weight loss. According to Jillian Micheals (Master Your Metabolism 2009) a key factor to keep in mind while undertaking this journey is your metabolism. Often, when communicating with clients about their undesired weight, the first reason they convey is that they have a slow metabolism. It is important for you to understand that your metabolism is not an incinerator that is supposed to burn everything you eat. On the contrary, what it is and what it does are two very different things. Your metabolism can be compared to a choir. It is a combination of hormones, cells, and molecules that work in synchronization to regulate the rate at which you burn calories.

It is these components that determine how the energy you consume through food will be used. Whether it's used now, stored as fat or used to build muscle, all of this would be determined by hormones that comprise your metabolism. The truth is our world has evolved rapidly. Everything is instant – food, fruits, vegetables anything you can think of is being manufactured in laboratories across the country, except for bodies! Well.

Some years ago, Adam and Eve, the first male and female, biblically speaking, hunted for food. They fished and farmed to survive. They ate nuts berries, fruits, meat from animals. Life was simple and good. Their bodies knew just what to do with that food they were eating but not today. You see our bodies are designed to recognize proteins, carbohydrates, fruits or vegetable your cells can identify it clearly and transport it through the blood stream to the necessary organs to aid in your bodies proper function. However, as a result of the instant age foods are not producing the natural way.

They are chemically injected which is ultimately changing its makeup thus causing the body to be confused as it relates to its purpose of being introduced to the body. It's a simple case of "identity theft" because everything is instant, the societal demand is greater than the supply. Food such as fruits and vegetables are not being allowed to come to full maturity, naturally. Animals are chemically injected to increase the rate of growth. We also come across food that is being produced at a high

28

rate of speed. For example, according to Jillian Michales (Master Your Metabolism 2009) High Fructose Corn Syrup which is a form of sugar that is cheaply manufactured to be profitable for big businesses. As their pockets get 'fat' so does your body.

It is imperative for you as you walk on this journey, to rule out all "offenders" that break this next principle. "If it does not grow on a tree, it's not for me, and if it did not have a mother, then I will not bother." Another easy way to remember this principle when reading the labels at the grocery store "If I cannot read it or understand what it is, don't eat it."

It is poison like these which are manufactured in laboratories that affect our hormones in a negative way; thus causing our bodies to store fat instead of burning it. Try telling your liver that high fructose corn syrup is food. It does not recognize the properties, and so your body is left to assume what it is and what to do with it. Nine times out of ten, it is not used, stored or disposed of correctly. It causes your body to compensate over for this foreign agent. High Fructose Corn Syrup just one example of poison that we have been consuming for years

According to High Fructose Corn Syrup https://en.wikipedia.org/wiki/High_fructose_corn_syr

up(n.d Wikipedia High-fructose corn syrup (HFCS) also called glucose-fructose isoglucose, and glucose-fructose syrup is a sweetener made from corn starch that has been processed by glucose isomerase to convert some of its glucose into fructose. HFCS was first marketed in the early 1970s by the Clinton Corn Processing Company, together with the Japanese research institute where the enzyme was discovered.

As a sweetener, HFCS is often compared to granulated sugar. Advantages of HFCS over granulated sugar include being easier to handle and being less expensive in some countries. However, there is also debate concerning whether HFCS presents greater health risks than other sweeteners. Use of HFCS peaked in the late 1990s; demand decreased due to public concern about a possible link between HFCS and metabolic diseases like obesity and diabetes.

Apart from comparisons between HFCS and table sugar, there is a strong scientific consensus that the over-consumption of added sugar, including HFCS, is a major health problem. Consuming added sugars, especially in the form of soft drinks, is strongly linked to obesity. The World Health Organization has recommended that people limit their consumption of added sugars to 10% of calories, but experts say that average consumption

I *am* the Lord who heals you. Exodus 15:26 NKJV

of empty calories in the United States is near twice that level. The U.S., HFCS is among the sweeteners that mostly replaced sucrose (table sugar) in the food industry. Factors include production quotas of domestic sugar, import tariff on foreign sugar, and subsidies for U.S. corn, raising the price of sucrose and lowering that of HFCS, making it cheapest for many sweetener applications. The relative sweetness of HFCS 55, used most commonly in soft drinks, is comparable to sucrose.

Because of its similar sugar profile and lower price, HFCS has been used illegally to "stretch" honey. Assays to detect adulteration with HFCS use differential scanning calorimetry and other advanced testing methods. So in other words, this stuff can kill you.

Next, we have the Grain. The next time while you're in the store doing your grocery shopping, you'd notice the words refined, enriched, and whole-grain written on grain products. These words describe the milling and making process, of grain products, and each term has different nutrition implications. According to Jillian Michaels (Master Your Metabolism 2009) Grains have three different key parts:

The Bran- which is the protective outer coating,

I *am* the Lord who heals you. Exodus 15:26 NKJV

which is rich in fiber and nutrients.

The Germ- which is the seed that grows into a wheat plant, so it's especially rich in vitamins and minerals to support new life.

Endosperm- contains starch and proteins. What makes whole-grain products so nutritious is that they contain much of the bran, germ, and the endosperm. The difference between white and wheat flour is significant – white bread is wheat bread stripped of all its naturally occurring nutrients. Whole grains haven't had the bran and germ removed by milling, making them excellent sources of fiber. Refined grains (white rice or flour) contain only the endosperm because they are stripped of the bran and germ. These items are then enriched by adding vitamins and minerals back after the milling process, but they still don't have the nutritional value or the fiber that whole grains contain.

According to Refined grains - Wikipedia, the free encyclopedia. (n.d.). Retrieved from https://en.wikipedia.org/wiki/Refined_grains , refined grains, in contrast to whole grains, refers to grain products consisting of grains or grain flours that have been significantly modified from their natural composition. The modification process generally involves the mechanical removal of bran and germ, either through grinding or selective sifting. Further refining includes mixing, bleaching, and brominating; additionally, thiamin, riboflavin, niacin, and iron are often added back into nutritionally enrich the product. Because the added nutrients represent a fraction of the nutrients removed, refined grains are considered nutritionally inferior to whole grains. However, for some grains the removal of fiber coupled with fine grinding results in a slightly higher availability of grain energy for use by the body. Furthermore, in the special case of maize, the process of nixtamalization (a chemical form of refinement) yields a considerable improvement in the bioavailability of niacin, thereby preventing pellagra in diets consisting largely of maize products.

I *am* the Lord who heals you. Exodus 15:26 NKJV

Step 4
Expel Key Offenders

Now that the foundation has is laid, we are now ready to erect the sides of the building. This list is the list that I followed according to Jillian Michaels Master your metabolism 2009) it is to serve as a recommendation, or a basic 'foundation' of products that you can remove from your diet by no means is it mandatory.

#1 offender - Hydrogenated Fats

The food process industry created hydrogenated fats; it is found in products like cookies, chips, crackers or bread. It helps food to have a longer shelf life and still maintains its freshness. Now think about it. Something is wrong when you can eat a product a year or two after it has been produced.

#2 offender - Refined Grains

Yes, grains are helpful and nutritional because thy come from the ground but once they are refined they no longer qualify. The process of refining a grain is done to extend the shelf life. The bran and the germ of the grain are removed, the fiber, vitamins, folic acid are stripped then restored by being enriched. The human body profits nothing from this process; only the pockets of human beings.

I *am* the Lord who heals you. Exodus 15:26 NKJV

#3 Offender - High Fructose Corn Syrup
High Fructose Corn Syrup is one of the cheapest sweeteners on the market. It helps food companies increase their profits and expands your waistline.

#4 Offender - Artificial Preservatives and Colors. Apart from the risk of consuming high fructose corn syrup and artificial sweeteners, benzoate salts are added to soda to prevent mold growth. Reports have found that this ingredient is poisonous when it sits in plastic bottles exposed to direct sunlight or heat. For example, a soda bottle.

#5 Offender - Glutamates
The most commonly talked about glutamate is monosodium glutamate or better known as MSG. Most people think MSG is a preservative; when in reality it's a flavor enhancer that is being exploited by the food industry. Reports have stated that high levels of free glutamates can 'mess' with your brain chemistry. Glutamates are a form of excitotoxin. Studies have shown that they can be devastating to the nervous system. Excitotoxins drive into the brain with relative ease, they excite brain cells and can rapidly cause permanent brain damage and eventual cell death

I *am* the Lord who heals you. Exodus 15:26 NKJV

Step 5
Empower you to Succeed

Now that we have exposed the truth and expelled some of the foods that have caused your hormones to become out of whack, we are going to enable and empower you to focus on food that helps to facilitate weight loss according to Jillian Michaels (Master Your Metabolism 2009)

#1 Power Food - Legumes
Yes, beans and other legumes are some of the richest sources of fiber which is vital for blood sugar control. Additionally, when you eat beans you feel fuller, store less fat, lower your cholesterol thus improve your body insulin sensitivity. Beans are also an excellent source of proteins and are rich in antioxidants.

#2 Power Food - the Allium Family
Garlic, onions, leeks chives, shallots, and scallions are great body detoxes. Garlic is my favorite. This family stimulates the body to produce an antioxidant that lives within each cell ready to fight free radicals. Garlic also helps to lower cholesterol.

#3 Power Food - Berries

Blackberries, blueberries, strawberries, yes berries. They are not fattening and have no caffeine. Berries also help to lower your blood sugar. Your insulin levels are critical to weight loss. Berries such as raspberries and strawberries are high in soluble fiber and make a sweet treat that works hard to help you lose weight.

#4 Power Food - Meat and Eggs

Yes, meat is a part of our success; but not just any meats, mainly those that are highly beneficial to our bodies. As we know, meat is a source of proteins and amino acids that are used to build muscle. Meats like wild Alaskan salmon; whole eggs provide proteins that increase your metabolic rate because it takes more energy to burn than if you ate carbs or fats.

#5 Power Food - Fruits and Vegetables

Yes, fruits and vegetables are the best. The more colorful your selection, the better. Fruits and vegetables are also high in fiber which is essential for balancing hormones. When people think of vegetables, they automatically think of greens. Yes, leafy greens are awesome, but they are not the only veggies that you should consume. You can also consume tomatoes that are high in fiber and gives you vitamin C.

I *am* the Lord who heals you. Exodus 15:26 NKJV

#6 Powerful Foods - Cruciferous and Dark Green Vegetables

Cruciferous and dark green vegetables are often referred to as super foods. Broccoli, cauliflower, and cabbage just to name a few are excellent sources of sulforaphane which is known to help the body to repair itself from damage. They also have a higher water and fiber content that leave you filled and increase your body's ability to burn fat. Dark leafy greens like spinach are also high in fiber and magnesium. The iron in spinach and Swiss chard is ideal for bringing oxygen to your muscles. The soluble fiber in dark green leafy veggies is known to help prevent inflammation. Spinach is also an excellent source of Omega 3 fats

#7 Power Food - Nuts and Seeds

Raw nuts and seeds are good snacks that help protect from heart disease, diabetes, and inflammation. Eating nuts like almonds pecans or walnuts are also high in fiber, antioxidant, omega 3 and so much more. Seeds also help reduce blood sugar spikes and maintain insulin level.

#8 Power Food - Whole Grains

Whole grains contribute to improving our hormone levels. Yes, whole grains not whole wheat. They improve our overall health. They are also an

I *am* the Lord who heals you. Exodus 15:26 NKJV

excellent source of antioxidants like oats and barley. Yes, I said barley helps to fight against heart disease and so much more. Whole grains do fall under the category of carbohydrates, but it is the kind that also helps us to eat less because they stimulate fat cells in our stomach. The high levels of fiber in whole grains also help us feel satisfied.

I *am* the Lord who heals you. Exodus 15:26 NKJV

Conclusion

Now that we have laid the foundation, taken you up the bell cost and pitched the roof, it's now time to apply the finishing touches.

At this point, your mind should be enlightened. You have rid yourself of all of the lies and now operating on the truth. You should also have a visualization of your destination i.e. the result you seek and the basic blueprint that I used to achieve my goals and are well on your way to achieving your individual goals based on the three (3) important steps we discussed: Expose; Expel; and Enable.

It has truly been my pleasure to share my journey with you and the tools that helped me to lose 100 pounds I pray it serves you well. "For with Christ nothing shall be impossibe".

Disclaimer

By no means, I am a doctor. The information given in this book should not replace the advice of your physician. Please communicate with your doctor before undertaking any changes. We are making suggestions relating

I *am* the Lord who heals you. Exodus 15:26 NKJV

Sample Shopping List

I *am* the Lord who heals you. Exodus 15:26 NKJV

Sample Shopping List

PROTEIN:

Egg Whites (6) 100 calories
Chicken Breast 110 calories
Turkey Breast 115 calories
95% Lean Grnd Beef 135 cal
Eye of Round 180 calories
Flank Steak 165 calories
Top sirloin 190 calories
Bison (buffalo) 110 calories
Venison (deer) 120 calories
1 can Tuna Fish in water 80 calories
Steak Lobster 95 calories
Crab 85 calories
Shrimp 110 calories
Scallops 95 calories
Orange Roughy 75 calories
Cod 85 calories
Flounder/Sole 90 calories
Sea Bass/Tilapia 100 calories
Halibut/Mahi-Mahi 110 calories

VEGETABLES:

Each serving is weighed in
 at 1 cup
Lettuce (any variety) 10 cal
umbers 20 calories

Tomatoes 35 calories
Celery 20 calories
Onions 65 calories
Spinach 10 calories
Chard 10 calories
Fennel 30 calories
Red Radishes 20 calories
Asparagus 30 calories
Cabbage 25 calories
Chicory 40 calories
Beet Greens 10 calories

DAIRY PROTEIN:

Make sure all products are "Fat Free"
Milk - 1 Cup (8 oz.) 90 calories
Yogurt (plain, non-fat) ¾ cup (6 oz.) 103 calories
Cottage Cheese (non-fat) ¾ cup (6 oz.) 100 calories

FRUIT:

Apple - 1 medium 74 calories
Orange - 1 medium 95 calories
Grapefruit - ¼ cup (sections) 85 calories
Strawberries - 1 cup (sliced) 50 calories
Blueberries - ½ cup (whole) 40 calories

STARCHES:

Melba Toast - (1) cracker 15 calories
Grissini Breadstick - (1) 15 calories
Saltine Crackers - (1) piece 20 cal
Wasa "Lite" Crackers - (1) piece 25-45 calories

I *am* the Lord who heals you. Exodus 15:26 NKJV

Black Coffee
No creamer (only 1 tablespoon
of fat free milk per day is
allowed for use in coffee/
tea; does not count as a dairy
selection).
Plain Black or Green Tea
Self–brewed. You may use
sweeteners; Stevia and
and plant base are
allowed. Aspartame, Sucralose
(Splenda) and regular sugar
are not allowed. You made add
flavor with a fresh lemon, lime
or orange only. No additional
added flavors or ingredients
in the tea packets or bags
including fruit, rosebuds,
roots, honey, etc. and do not
consume pre-bottled teas.

Spices / Seasonings:

You can use any spice you
want, just be sure it doesn't
contain sugar or starch. Salt
and pepper are allowed.
Read the ingredients of
everything you consume, even
a minor intake of something
that is not allowed can affect
your results

Chewing Gum:
You can have gum, but be
sure it is fl avored ONLY with
Xylitol (a natural sweetener).
Most brands use Aspartame,
which is not allowed.

I *am* the Lord who heals you. Exodus 15:26 NKJV

Sample 7 Day Meal Plan
Base on 1200 calories

DAY ONE
Breakfast Egg white omelet with spinach and tomatoes
Lunch Grilled chicken with cold chicory salad
Snack Celery sticks + savory dill dressing
Dinner Poached halibut + steamed asparagus
Dessert Sugar-free Gelatin

DAY TWO
Breakfast Nonfat Greek yogurt + 1 orange
Lunch Tilapia or Tuna (oil free, in water)
Snack Fruit w/ warm vanilla sauce
Dinner Chinese Chicken Salad
Dessert Fat-free frozen Strawberry sorbe

DAY THREE
Breakfast Egg whites
Lunch Mongolian beef with cabbage
Snack Lemonade
Dinner Tilapia with herbs
Dessert Sugar-Free Applesauce with cinnamon

DAY FOUR
Breakfast Strawberry smoothie
Lunch Chinese chicken salad
Snack Tomato basil soup
Dinner Creole Shrimp + steamed spinach
Dessert Fruit with warm vanilla sauce

I *am* the Lord who heals you. Exodus 15:26 NKJV

DAY FIVE
Breakfast Nonfat cottage cheese + 1 orange
Lunch Shrimp cocktail + ceviche
Snack Melba toast with strawberry jam
Dinner Baked Cajun chicken + saffron
cabbage
Dessert Apple Chips

DAY SIX
Breakfast Egg whites with allowed veggies of
your choice
Lunch Curried shrimp with tomatoes &
Indian rice
Snack Melba toast with strawberry jam
Dinner Pepper crusted steak + garlic spinach
Dessert Chilled Sugar-Free Orange Pops

DAY SEVEN
Breakfast ½ Grapefruit
Lunch Breaded chicken cutlets + cucumber
salad
Snack N/A Bloody Hot Thin Mary
Dinner Creole Gumbo + grilled asparagus
Dessert Zucchini Bread

I *am* the Lord who heals you. Exodus 15:26 NKJV

References

I *am* the Lord who heals you. Exodus 15:26 NKJV

References

Page 1-26
The Bible (King James Version) //www.biblegateway.com

Page 19-20
Harris–Benedict equation - Wikipedia, the free encyclopedia
https://en.wikipedia.org/wiki/Harris–Benedict_equationWikipedia
https://en.wikipedia.org/wiki/Basal_metabolic_rate (n.d)

Page 22
Counting calories: Get back to weight-loss basics - Mayo Clinic
www.mayoclinic.org/healthy-lifestyle/weight-loss/.../calories/art-
20048065Mayo Clinic (April 11, 2015)

The Obesity Society facts about obesity
http://www.obesity.org/resources/facts-about-obesity (last
updated April 2016)

Michaels, J., Mariska V., A. "Jillian Michaels Master Your
Metabolism," (2009)

Page 25-26
High Fructose Corn Syrup
https://en.wikipedia.org/wiki/High_fructose_corn_syrup(n.d)

Bouchez, C. " Make the most of your Metabolism,"

www.webmd.com (February 24, 2006)

Page 30
High Fructose Corn Syrup

I *am* the Lord who heals you. Exodus 15:26 NKJV

https://en.wikipedia.org/wiki/High_fructose_corn_syrup(n.d)

5 Reasons High Fructose Corn Syrup Will Kill You - Dr. Mark Hyman
drhyman.com/blog/.../5-reasons-high-fructose-corn-syrup-will-kill-you

Page
Refined grains https://en.wikipedia.org/wiki/Refined_grains (last updated March 24, 2016)

Page 32

What are hydrogenated fats? - The World's Healthiest Foods
www.whfoods.com/genpage. (n.d.)

Consumer Report "Benzene in Soft Drinks. Consumer Repots October 2006
www.consumerreports.org

http://www.honeycolony.com/article/excitotoxins-the-fda-approved-way-to-damage-your-brain/ (Anonymous Jun 22, 2015)

Michaels, J., Mariska V., A., "Jillian Michaels Master Your Metabolism," (2009)

Page 37
the nal formula for your Resolution to weight loss. The. (n.d.). Retrieved   from
https://totallifechanges.zendesk.com/hc/en-us/article_attachments/202896987/reso

JOIN OUR FACEBOOK COMMUNITY

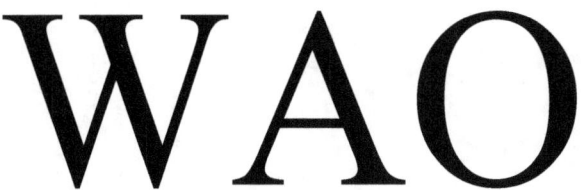

THE WAR AGAINST OBESITY THE CAUSE

I *am* the Lord who heals you. Exodus 15:26 NKJV

I *am* the Lord who heals you. Exodus 15:26 NKJV

www.ingramcontent.com/pod-product-compliance
Lightning Source LLC
Chambersburg PA
CBHW062022280526
45787CB00005B/2194